THE 2020
SIRTFOOD
DIET
WITH BONUS RECIPES

A HEALTHY DIET PLAN TO ACHIEVE SEVEN-POUND WEIGHT LOSS IN SEVEN DAYS WITHOUT STARVING

SANDRA J. PARKER

Goodwater Publishing
279 Stoney Lane
Dallas, TX 75212
Texas
USA

Copyright © 2020 Sandra J. Parker

CONTENTS

INTRODUCTION

Weight loss is an issue constantly on many people's minds. Almost everyone wants to be slim and toned, but the reality is that it is far easier to gain weight than to lose it. Healthy weight loss can be achieved by following a healthy weight loss diet. This book introduces Sirtfood diet, a simple healthy way of eating that promises a seven-pound weight loss in seven days without losing muscle mass. It is healthy because you eat and lose weight without feeling hungry.

The Sirtfood diet is built around natural compounds found in fruits and vegetables called polyphenols. These polyphenols mimic the effects of fasting and exercise by activating proteins in the bodies called sirtuins. The sirtuins also known as SIRTs, or silent information regulators when activated help the body to burn fat, increase muscle mass, and improve your health. In simpler terms, Sirtfoods stimulate sirtuin genes, which help to protect the cells in the body from inflammation or death through illness (anti-aging effect). They also help to improve memory function, control blood sugar level, and reduce the risk of chronic disease.

The Sirtfood diet introduces a list of foods and beverages that function as the best sirtuin activators and they include but not limited to the following:

- Apple
- Arugula (rocket)

- Bird's eye chili (peppers)
- Blueberries
- Buckwheat
- Capers
- Celery
- Citrus fruit
- Coffee
- Dark chocolate (85% cocoa)
- Extra-virgin olive oil
- Garlic
- Ginger
- Kale
- Lovage
- Matcha green tea
- Medjool dates
- Parsley
- Red chicory
- Red onions
- Red wine
- Soy
- Strawberries
- Turmeric
- Walnuts

SIRTFOOD HEALTH BENEFITS

Sirtfoods are healthy foods that are rich in sirtuin activators which help you lose weight. The consumption of balanced sirtfoods helps to boosts metabolism and also slows down the aging process. Some of the potential health benefits of the sirtfoods are considered here and they include the following:

Extra-virgin Olive Oil

Extra-virgin olive oil contains the major sirtuin-activating nutrients called oleuropein and hydroxytyrosol. Some of its health benefits include:

1. Aids weight loss: It helps in achieving and sustaining a long-lasting weight loss result.
2. Improves sex life: It helps in the circulation of blood to all parts of the body especially the erogenous zones.
3. Prevents type 2 diabetes: Using extra-virgin olive oil as part of sirtfood diet helps to regulate and balance the body sugar level, thus preventing diabetes.
4. Pain relief: Extra-virgin olive oil contains anti-inflammatory properties which help to impact several chronic diseases in the body.

5. Immune system boost: Extra-virgin olive oil contains antioxidants that are good for protecting the body's immune system by becoming resistant to infections.

6. Improves brain health: Extra-virgin olive oil could potentially reduce the risk of Alzheimer's disease and age-related dementia.

7. Pregnancy aid: Not only can olive oil application assist in avoiding stretch marks, consuming extra-virgin olive oil while pregnant may improve your child's psychomotor reflexes and more.

Bird's-Eye Chilies

The Sirtfood Bird's-Eye Chilies (sometimes referred to as 'Thai chilies') contain the major sirtuin-activating nutrients luteolin and myricetin. It also contains capsaicin, which is a chemical compound that results in the burning sensation of the mouth, throat, and stomach upon ingestion and its effects vary among individuals. If you are not used to spicy food, it is recommended you start with half the chili amount stated in the recipe, as well as deseeding your chili before use. You can adjust the heat to your preference throughout the diet.

The health benefits of the Bird's eye chilies include:

1. Significant in weight loss: Upon ingestion of Bird's eye chilies, they change the body's metabolism by increasing the body temperature. To bring back the body to the original temperature, the body would burn more calories by using the unused fats stored in various parts of the body.

2. Aids digestion: It helps in improving digestion by increasing the production flows of enzymes and also gastric acid which speeds up the intestinal tract movement.

3. Lowers blood pressure: Capsaicin found in the bird's eye chili helps to clear the flow of blood throughout the whole body so that it won't pile up and block the arteries of the heart.

4. Natural pain relief: It has anti-inflammatory agents which makes it useful in the alleviation of pains caused by arthritis, rheumatism, osteoarthritis, psoriasis, shingles, and diabetic neuropathy by tuning down sensory receptors.

Red Wine

Red wine contains the major sirtuin-activating nutrients resveratrol and piceatannol. Here are some of the health benefits of red wine when taken in moderation. Drinking one to two glasses of red wine per day may be considered to be *moderate drinking*.

1. Reduced risk of cancer: Consuming red wine in moderation helps to reduce the risk of several cancers such as colon, ovary, and prostate cancers.

2. Reduced risk of stroke: Moderate consumption of red wine helps to prevent blood clotting. Red wine acts as a natural blood thinner, breaking up any blood clots that could lead to a stroke.

3. Lowers cholesterol: consumption of red wine in moderation helps to decrease the low-density lipoproteins, LDL (bad cholesterol) and increase the high-density lipoproteins, HDL (good cholesterol) in the body.

4. Promotes longevity: The resveratrol present in red wine helps to reduce some of the damage caused by the natural aging process, particularly as it concerns the heart.

Buckwheat

Buckwheat is often referred to as a pseudocereal and it's not in any way related to wheat at all. Pseudocereals are seeds that are consumed as cereal grains but don't grow on grasses. Buckwheat can be made into noodles, pancakes, porridge, and a variety of baked foods.

Here are some of the health benefits of this pseudocereal sirtfood:

1. Aids in weight loss: Buckwheat is low in calories compared with barley and wheat. As such, it enhances insulin sensitivity of the body and reduces the accumulation of fat in the bloodstream.

2. High content of fiber: Buckwheat is rich in fiber and as such it's good for those with constipation. It also helps to decrease the risk of colon cancer

3. Improved heart health: This pseudocereal helps to stabilize blood pressure and reduces the bad cholesterol level in the body. This in return maintains the overall heart health.

4. Stabilizes blood sugar: The buckwheat has a known slow rate of breakdown and absorption of carbohydrates into the bloodstream. This results in the gradual flow of energy and the prevention of a sudden spike in blood sugar.

5. Prevent gallstones: Consumption of buckwheat helps to prevent gallstones in both men and women. This is as a result of the buckwheat speeding up the intestinal transmits time (the speed at which food moves through the intestine and reduces the release of bile acids), which is one of the contributing factors in gallstone formation.

Matcha Green Tea

Matcha, which is one of the popular sirtfoods available in coffee shops, is a type of tea that's far less processed than regular green tea. The leaves are never heated and are kept under shade to preserve the natural nutrients found in the leaves. Here are some of the health benefits of matcha green tea:

1. High antioxidant agent: Matcha contains a very high level of an antioxidant agent called EGCG (epigallocatechin gallate), which is believed to have cancer-fighting and improved aging effects on the body.

2. Supports weight loss: Matcha helps increase metabolism and fat burning, both of which aids weight loss.

3. Provides calmness and improves focus: Matcha is rich in L-Theanine, a rare amino acid that promotes a state of relaxation and well-being of the body by acting upon the brains functioning. L-Theanine also helps to inhibit any possible side-effects from caffeine. In other words, a bowl of matcha promotes concentration and clarity of mind without any of the nervous energy found in coffee.

4. Effective and natural detoxifier: Matcha leaves are shade-grown and, as such, they produce extra chlorophyll in their leaves. The chlorophyll has powerful detoxifying properties including the ability to naturally eliminate chemicals and heavy metals from the body.

Medjool Dates

Medjool dates, which are often informally known as the *king of dates*, are edible sweet fruits that come from the date palm tree. They're often sold dried but not dehydrated, making them soft and sticky. Their sugars become more concentrated as they dry, which further increases their sweetness.

Here are some of the health benefits of consuming Medjool dates:

1. Relieves and prevents constipation: Medjool dates have high fiber content and as such, they help promote healthy digestion and bowel movement regularity; thereby preventing constipation.
2. Lowers cholesterol level: Medjool dates which are high in dietary fiber can lower the high-density lipoproteins (LDL) cholesterol in the blood. LDL is a

type of fat-like substance responsible for such conditions as heart disease and stroke.

3. Prevents and relieves constipation: Medjool dates have high levels of soluble fiber, which keep bowel movements regular by adding bulk to stool and helping it move faster through the intestines.

4. Energy booster: Medjool dates contain natural sugars like sucrose, glucose, and fructose, more than many other fruits. These sugars are easily processed and utilized by the body for energy.

Dark Chocolate (85% cocoa)

Dark chocolate is a bar of rich, bitter chocolate that is typically made of cocoa solids, sugar, and cocoa butter (and doesn't contain any milk). The percentage of cocoa affects flavor and bitterness. The darker the chocolate, the better it is. Here are some of the health benefits of eating dark chocolate:

1. Promotes weight loss: Eating a bit of dark chocolate before or after meals triggers hormones that signal to the brain you're full and this can last for a longer time. They are also packed with monounsaturated fatty acids that are known to boost your metabolism and burn fat.

2. Lowers Cholesterol: Dark chocolate raises high-density lipoproteins (HDL). At the same time, it lowers the low-density lipoproteins (LDL), which when in high amounts can clog arteries.

3. Lowers blood pressure: High magnesium content in dark chocolates helps in lowering blood pressure. Consuming them increases nitric oxide level which is a naturally occurring substance in our body that acts on small receptors in our blood vessels and helps them dilate. Thereby, lowering overall blood pressure.

SIRTFOOD DIET PLAN

The Sirtfood diet plan has two phases and is meant to last for three weeks. The first phase is broken into two parts: the first three days and the last four days. During the first phase, you are expected to lose about seven pounds in seven days. While the second phase which is called the *maintenance period* is meant to last for two weeks. The second phase is intended to help you lose weight steadily. The two phases can be repeated whenever you feel like losing weight afterward. However, it is advisable to continue drinking the sirtfood green juice every day and incorporating sirtfoods regularly into your meals after completing these phases. In this way, the Sirtfood diet becomes more of a lifestyle change than a one-time diet.

First Phase

This book presents a complete seven-day meal plan with each day's easy-to-follow, delicious recipes. It's noteworthy that you are not allowed to drink any alcohol during this phase, but you can drink water, tea, coffee, and green tea freely. The first phase meal plan recipes are based on the two distinct stages as thus:

(Days 1–3):

- Calories intake per day should be limited to 1,000 calories during the first three days of the diet

- Three glasses of sirtfood green juice should be taken on each day

- Eat one full meal rich in sirtfood per day

- 10-20g dark chocolate(85% cocoa) is permitted

(Days 4–7):

- Calories intake per day during the last four days of this phase should be increased to 1,500 calories
- Two glasses of sirtfood green juice should be taken on each day

- Eat two full meal rich in sirtfood per day

- 10-20g dark chocolate(85% cocoa) is permitted

Second Phase

The second phase of this dietary plan involves packing together rich sirtfoods. During this second phase, you are allowed to drink red wine, but in moderation (the recommendation is 2-3 glasses of red wine per week), as well as water, tea, coffee, and green tea. This book puts together a rich seven-day sirtfood diet meal plan to follow with a repetition to complete the fourteen days of the second phase.

The second phase meal plan recipes are based on the directives below:

- Eat three balanced meals rich in sirtfoods for the remaining two weeks

- One glass of sirtfood green juice should be taken on each day.

- To maintain your results, it's recommended that you still include lots of sirtfoods in your diet, while sticking to mostly balanced, plant-based meals.

21-Day Sirtfood Diet Guide

The recipes for cooking the meals on this guide are on pages 21 – 63. You can find bonus recipes on pages 64 – 100 to help you alternate the stipulated meals in this guide.

WEEK 1
FIRST PHASE (SEVEN-POUNDS LOSS PERIOD)

	BREAKFAST	LUNCH	DINNER
DAY 1	1 glass of Sirtfood green juice.	2 glasses of Sirtfood green juice.	Recipe 1: **Asian King Prawn Stir Fry with Buckwheat Noodles.** 10-20g dark chocolate (85% cocoa) is

			permitted to be taken after dinner if you so desire.
DAY 2	1 glass of Sirtfood green juice.	2 glasses of Sirtfood green juice.	Recipe 2: **Kale and Red Onion Dhal with Buckwheat.** 10-20g dark chocolate (85% cocoa) is permitted to be taken after dinner if you so desire.
DAY 3	1 glass of Sirtfood green juice.	2 glasses of Sirtfood green juice.	Recipe 3: **Aromatic Chicken with Kale, Buckwheat, and Salsa.** 10-20g dark chocolate (85% cocoa) is permitted to be taken after dinner if you so desire.
DAY 4	1 glass of Sirtfood green juice.	Recipe 4: **Sirt Muesli**.	Recipe 5: **Tuscan Bean Stew with**

	BREAKFAST	LUNCH	DINNER
		1 glass of Sirtfood green juice.	**Buckwheat.**
DAY 5	1 glass of Sirtfood green juice.	Recipe 6: **Strawberry buckwheat tabbouleh.** 1 glass of Sirtfood green juice.	Recipe 7: **Miso marinated baked cod with stir-fried greens and sesame.**
DAY 6	2 glasses of Sirtfood green juice.	Recipe 8: **Green Juice Salad.**	Recipe 9: **Chargrilled beef with red wine jus, and herb roasted potatoes.**
DAY 7	2 glasses of Sirtfood green juice.	Recipe 10: **Sirtfood omelet with bacon.**	Recipe 11: **Baked Chicken Breast with Walnut and Parsley Pesto and Red Onion Salad.**

WEEK 2
SECOND PHASE (MAINTENANCE PERIOD)

	BREAKFAST	LUNCH	DINNER
DAY 8	Recipe 12: **Blueberry smoothie.**	Recipe 13: **Sirtfood Shakshuka.**	Recipe 14: **Chicken Escalope with sage, caper and**

			parsley and spiced cauliflower 'couscous'.

1 glass of Sirtfood green juice.

(to be taken at any time of the day as you chose)

DAY 9	Recipe 15: **Apple Pancakes with Blackcurrant Compote.**	Recipe 16: **Coronation chicken salad.**	Recipe 17: **Prawn Arrabbiata.**

1 glass of Sirtfood green juice.

(to be taken at any time of the day as you chose)

DAY 10	Recipe 4: **Sirt Muesli.**	Recipe 18: **Buckwheat pasta salad.**	Recipe 19: **Beef Bourguignon stew with mashed potatoes and vegetables.**

1 glass of Sirtfood green juice.

(to be taken at any time of the day as you chose)

DAY 11	Recipe 20: **Kale and Blackcurrant Smoothie.**	Recipe 21: **Waldorf Salad.**	Recipe 22: **Chili Con Carne with Buckwheat.**

1 glass of Sirtfood green juice.

(to be taken at any time of the day as you chose)

DAY	Recipe 23:	Recipe 6:	Recipe 24:

| 12 | Blueberry Banana Pancakes with Chunky Apple Compote and Golden Turmeric Latte. | Strawberry buckwheat tabbouleh. | Sirtfood Braised Puy Lentils. |

1 glass of Sirtfood green juice.

(to be taken at any time of the day as you chose)

| DAY 13 | Recipe 25: **Green Tea Smoothie.** | Recipe 26: **Salmon Sirt Super Salad.** | Recipe 27: **Chinese –style Pork with Pak Choi.** |

1 glass of Sirtfood green juice.

(to be taken at any time of the day as you chose)

| DAY 14 | Recipe 28: **Buckwheat Pancakes with Strawberries, Dark Chocolate Sauce, and Crushed Walnuts.** | Recipe 29: **Sesame Chicken Salad.** | Recipe 30: **Chickpea, Quinoa, and Turmeric Curry.** |

1 glass of Sirtfood green juice.

(to be taken at any time of the day as you chose)

WEEK 3

	BREAKFAST	**LUNCH**	**DINNER**
DAY 15	Recipe 12: **Blueberry smoothie.**	Recipe 13: **Sirtfood Shakshuka.**	Recipe 14: **Chicken Escalope with sage, caper and**

parsley and spiced cauliflower 'couscous'.

1 glass of Sirtfood green juice.

(to be taken at any time of the day as you chose)

DAY 16	Recipe 15: **Apple Pancakes with Blackcurrant Compote.**	Recipe 16: **Coronation chicken salad.**	Recipe 17: **Prawn Arrabbiata.**

1 glass of Sirtfood green juice.

(to be taken at any time of the day as you chose)

DAY 17	Recipe 4: **Sirt Muesli.**	Recipe 18: **Buckwheat pasta salad.**	Recipe 19: **Beef Bourguignon stew with mashed potatoes and vegetables.**

1 glass of Sirtfood green juice.

(to be taken at any time of the day as you chose)

DAY 18	Recipe 20: **Kale and Blackcurrant Smoothie.**	Recipe 21: **Waldorf Salad.**	Recipe 22: **Chili Con Carne with Buckwheat.**

1 glass of Sirtfood green juice.

(to be taken at any time of the day as you chose)

DAY	Recipe 23:	Recipe 6:	Recipe 24:

| 19 | Blueberry Banana Pancakes with Chunky Apple Compote and Golden Turmeric Latte. | Strawberry buckwheat tabbouleh. | Sirtfood Braised Puy Lentils. |

1 glass of Sirtfood green juice.
(to be taken at any time of the day as you chose)

| DAY 20 | Recipe 25: **Green Tea Smoothie.** | Recipe 26: **Salmon Sirt Super Salad.** | Recipe 27: **Chinese –style Pork with Pak Choi.** |

1 glass of Sirtfood green juice.
(to be taken at any time of the day as you chose)

| DAY 21 | Recipe 28: **Buckwheat Pancakes with Strawberries, Dark Chocolate Sauce, and Crushed Walnuts.** | Recipe 29: **Sesame Chicken Salad.** | Recipe 30: **Chickpea, Quinoa, and Turmeric Curry.** |

1 glass of Sirtfood green juice.
(to be taken at any time of the day as you chose)

SIRTFOOD DIET RECIPES

Sirtfood Diet Green Juice

Prep time 5 minutes

Total time 5 minutes

Serves 1

Ingredients:

- 75g kale
- 30g rocket
- 5g parsley
- 2 celery stalks
- ½ medium green apple
- 1 cm ginger
- Juice of ½ lemon
- ½ teaspoon matcha green tea powder

Method:

1. Juice all the ingredients apart from the lemon and the matcha green tea.
2. Squeeze the lemon juice into the green juice by hand.
3. Pour a small amount of green juice into a glass and stir in the matcha. Add the rest of the green juice into the glass and stir it again.
4. Drink straight away or save for later.

Recipe 1: Asian King Prawn Stir Fry with Buckwheat Noodles

Prep time 5 minutes

Cook time 15 minutes

Total time 20 minutes

Serves 4

Ingredients:

- 300g buckwheat noodles (100% buckwheat preferable)
- 2 tablespoons extra-virgin olive oil
- 1 red onion, sliced thinly
- 2 stalks of celery, sliced
- 100g kale, roughly chopped
- 100g green beans, chopped
- 3cm fresh ginger, grated
- 3 garlic clove, grated or finely chopped
- 1 bird's eye chili, seeds removed and chopped finely
- 600g shelled raw king prawns, deveined
- 2 tablespoons tamari (use soy sauce if you are not avoiding gluten)
- 5g parsley or lovage, chopped

Method:

1. Cook the noodles for 3-5 minutes or until they are done to your liking. Drain, rinse in cold water. Drizzle over a little olive oil, mix and set aside.

2. While the noodles are cooking, prepare the rest of the ingredients.

3. In a large frying pan, fry the red onion and celery in a little olive oil over a gentle heat for 3 minutes until soft, then add the kale and green beans and fry over medium-high heat for 3 minutes.

4. Turn the heat down again and add the ginger, garlic, chili, and prawns. Fry for 2-3 minutes until the prawns are hot all the way through.

5. Add the noodles, tamari/soy sauce, and cook for 1 more minute until the noodles are warm again. Sprinkle with parsley or lovage and serve.

Recipe 2: Kale and Red Onion Dhal with Buckwheat

Prep time 5 minutes

Cook time 25 minutes

Total time 30 minutes

Serves 4

Ingredients:

- 1 tablespoon olive oil

- 1 small red onion, sliced

- 3 garlic cloves, grated or crushed

- 2 cm ginger, grated

- 1 bird's eye chili, deseeded and finely chopped

- 2 teaspoons turmeric

- 2 teaspoons garam masala

- 160g red lentils

- 400ml coconut milk

- 200ml water

- 100g kale or spinach would be a great alternative

- 160g buckwheat

Method:

1. Put the olive oil in a large, deep saucepan and add the sliced onion. Cook on low heat, with the lid on for 5 minutes until softened.

2. Add the garlic, ginger, and chili and cook for 1 more minute.

3. Add the turmeric, garam masala, and a splash of water and cook for 1 more minute.

4. Add the red lentils, coconut milk, and 200ml water (do this simply by half filling the coconut milk can with water and tipping it into the saucepan).

5. Mix everything thoroughly and cook for 20 minutes over a gentle heat with the lid on. Stir occasionally and add a little more water if the dhal starts to stick.

6. After 20 minutes add the kale, stir thoroughly and replace the lid, cook for a further 5 minutes (1-2 minutes if you use spinach instead!)

7. About 15 minutes before the curry is ready, place the buckwheat in a medium saucepan and add plenty of boiling water. Bring the water back to the boil and cook for 10 minutes (or a little longer if you prefer your buckwheat softer. Drain the buckwheat in a sieve and serve with the dhal.

Recipe 3: Aromatic Chicken with Kale, Buckwheat, and Salsa

Serves 1

Ingredients:

- 120g skinless, boneless chicken breast
- 2 teaspoons ground turmeric
- Juice of ¼ lemon
- 1 tablespoon extra-virgin olive oil
- 50g kale, chopped
- 20g red onion, sliced
- 1 teaspoon chopped fresh ginger
- 50g buckwheat

For the Salsa

- 1 medium tomato (130g)
- 1 bird's eye chili, finely chopped
- 1 tablespoon capers, finely chopped
- 2 tablespoons (5g) parsley, finely chopped
- Juice of ¼ lemon

Method:

1. To make the salsa, remove the eye from the tomato and chop it very finely, taking care to keep as much of the liquid as possible. Mix with the chili, capers, parsley, and lemon juice. You could put everything in a blender, but the result is a little different.
2. Heat the oven to 220°C.
3. Marinate the chicken breast in 1 teaspoon of the turmeric, the lemon juice, and a little oil. Leave for 5 to 10 minutes.
4. Heat an ovenproof frying pan until hot, then add the marinated chicken and cook for a minute or so on each side, until pale golden, then transfer to the oven (place on a baking tray if your pan isn't ovenproof) for 8 to 10 minutes or until cooked through. Remove from the oven, cover with foil, and leave to rest for 5 minutes before serving.
5. Meanwhile, cook the kale in a steamer for 5 minutes. Fry the red onions and the ginger in a little oil, until

soft but not browned, then add the cooked kale and
fry for another minute.

6. Cook the buckwheat according to the package
   instructions with the remaining teaspoon of turmeric.
   Serve alongside the chicken, vegetables, and salsa.

Recipe 4: Sirt Muesli

Ingredients:

- 20g buckwheat flakes
- 10g buckwheat puffs
- 15g coconut flakes or desiccated coconut
- 40g Medjool dates, pitted and chopped
- 15g walnuts, chopped
- 10g cocoa nibs
- 100g strawberries, hulled and chopped
- 100g plain Greek yogurt (or vegan alternative, such as
  soya or coconut yogurt)

Method:

1. Mix all of the above ingredients (leave out the
   strawberries and yogurt if not serving straight away).

Recipe 5: Tuscan Bean Stew with Buckwheat

Ingredients:

- 1 tablespoon extra-virgin olive oil
- 50g red onion, finely chopped
- 30g carrot, peeled and finely chopped
- 30g celery, trimmed and finely chopped
- 1 garlic clove, finely chopped
- ½ bird's eye chili, finely chopped (optional)
- 1 teaspoon herbes de Provence
- 200ml vegetable stock
- 1 x 400g tin chopped Italian tomatoes
- 1 teaspoon tomato purée
- 200g tinned mixed beans
- 50g kale, roughly chopped
- 1 tablespoon roughly chopped parsley
- 40g buckwheat

Method:

1. Place the oil in a medium saucepan over low–medium heat and gently fry the onion, carrot, celery, garlic, chili (if using) and herbs, until the onion is soft but not colored.

2. Add the vegetable stock, tomatoes and tomato purée and bring to the boil. Add the beans and simmer for 30 minutes.

3. Add the kale and cook for another 5–10 minutes, until tender, then add the parsley.

4. Meanwhile, cook the buckwheat according to the packet instructions, drain and then serve with the stew.

Recipe 6: Strawberry buckwheat tabbouleh

Serves 1

Ingredients:

- 50g buckwheat
- 1 tablespoon ground turmeric
- 80g avocado
- 65g tomato
- 20g red onion
- 25g Medjool dates, pitted
- 1 tablespoon capers
- 30g parsley
- 100g strawberries, hulled
- 1 tablespoon extra-virgin olive oil
- Juice of ½ lemon
- 30g arugula

Method:

1. Cook the buckwheat with the turmeric according to
    the package instructions. Drain and set aside to cool.
2. Finely chop the avocado, tomato, red onion, dates,
    capers, and parsley and mix with the cool buckwheat.
3. Slice the strawberries and gently mix into the salad
    with the oil and lemon juice. Serve on a bed of
    arugula.

Recipe 7: Miso marinated baked cod with stir-fried greens and sesame

Serves 1

Ingredients:

- 20g miso
- 1 tablespoon mirin
- 1 tablespoon extra-virgin olive oil
- 200g skinless cod fillet
- 20g red onion, sliced
- 40g celery, sliced
- 2 garlic clove, finely chopped
- 1 bird's eye chili, finely chopped
- 1 teaspoon finely chopped fresh ginger
- 60g green beans
- 50g kale, roughly chopped
- 1 teaspoon sesame seeds

- 5g parsley, roughly chopped
- 1 tablespoon tamari (or soy sauce, if not avoiding gluten)
- 40g buckwheat
- 1 teaspoon ground turmeric

Method:

1. Mix the miso, mirin, and 1 teaspoon of the oil. Rub all over the cod and leave to marinate for 30 minutes.
2. Heat the oven to 220°C.
3. Bake the cod for 10 minutes.
4. Meanwhile, heat a large frying pan or wok with the remaining oil. Add the onion and stir-fry for a few minutes, then add the celery, garlic, chili, ginger, green beans, and kale. Toss and fry until the kale is tender and cooked through. You may need to add a little water to the pan to aid the cooking process.
5. Cook the buckwheat according to the packet instructions together with the turmeric for 3 minutes.
6. Add the sesame seeds, parsley, and tamari to the stir-fry and serve with the buckwheat and fish.

Recipe 8: Green Juice Salad

Prep time 10 minutes

Total time 10 minutes

Serves 1

Ingredients:

- Juice of ½ lemon
- 1 cm ginger grated
- Salt and pepper to taste
- 1 tablespoon olive oil
- 2 handfuls kale sliced
- 1 handful rocket
- 1 tablespoon parsley
- 2 celery stalks sliced
- ½ green apple sliced
- 6 walnut halves

Method:

1. Put the lemon juice, ginger, salt, pepper, and olive oil in a jam jar and shake to combine.
2. Place the kale in a large bowl and pour over the dressing. Massage the dressing into the kale for 1 minute.
3. Add all the other ingredients and mix thoroughly.

Recipe 9: Chargrilled beef with red wine jus, and herb-roasted potatoes

Ingredients:

- 100g potatoes, peeled and cut into 2cm dice
- 1 tablespoon extra-virgin olive oil
- 5g parsley, finely chopped
- 50g red onion, sliced into rings
- 50g kale, sliced
- 1 garlic clove, finely chopped
- 120–150g x 3.5cm-thick beef fillet steak or 2cm-thick sirloin steak
- 40ml red wine
- 150ml beef stock
- 1 teaspoon tomato purée
- 1 teaspoon cornflour, dissolved in 1 tablespoon water

Method:

1. Heat the oven to 220°C.
2. Place the potatoes in a saucepan of boiling water, bring back to the boil and cook for 4–5 minutes, then drain. Place in a roasting tin with 1 teaspoon of the oil and roast in the hot oven for 35–45 minutes. Turn the potatoes every 10 minutes to ensure even cooking. When cooked, remove from the oven, sprinkle with the chopped parsley and mix well.

3. Fry the onion in 1 teaspoon of the oil over medium heat for 5–7 minutes, until soft and nicely caramelized. Keep warm. Steam the kale for 2–3 minutes then drain. Fry the garlic gently in ½ teaspoon of oil for 1 minute, until soft but not colored. Add the kale and fry for a further 1–2 minutes, until tender. Keep warm.

4. Heat an ovenproof frying pan over high heat until smoking. Coat the meat in ½ a teaspoon of the oil and fry in the hot pan over medium-high heat according to how you like your meat done. If you like your meat medium it would be better to sear the meat and then transfer the pan to an oven set at 220°C and finish the cooking that way for the prescribed times.

5. Remove the meat from the pan and set aside to rest. Add the wine to the hot pan to bring up any meat residue. Bubble to reduce the wine by half, until syrupy and with a concentrated flavor.

6. Add the stock and tomato purée to the steak pan and bring to the boil, then add the cornflour paste to thicken your sauce, adding it a little at a time until you have your desired consistency. Stir in any of the juices from the rested steak and serve with the roasted potatoes, kale, onion rings, and red wine sauce.

Recipe 10: Sirtfood Omelet with Bacon

Serves 1

Ingredients:

- 1 teaspoon Extra-virgin Olive oil
- 35g red endive, thinly sliced
- 5g Parsley, finely chopped
- 1 Teaspoon Turmeric
- 50gm (2 ounces) Sliced Streaky Bacon (or 2 smoked or regular rashers, according to your taste)
- 3 Medium Eggs

Method:

1. Heat a nonstick frying pan. Cut the bacon into thin strips and cook over high heat until crispy. You do not need to add any oil, there is enough fat in the bacon to cook it. Remove from the pan and place on a paper towel to drain any excess fat. Wipe the pan clean.
2. Whisk the eggs and mix with the endive, parsley, and turmeric.
3. Chop the cooked bacon into cubes and stir through the eggs.
4. Heat the oil in the frying pan—the pan should be hot but not smoking. Add the egg mixture and, using a spatula, move it around the pan to start to cook the

egg. Keep the bits of cooked egg moving and swirl the raw egg around the pan until the omelet level is even.

5. Reduce the heat and let the omelet firm up. Ease the spatula around the edges and fold the omelet in half or roll up and serve.

Recipe 11: Baked Chicken Breast with Walnut and Parsley Pesto and Red Onion Salad

Prep time 15 minutes

Cook time 30 minutes

Total time 45 minutes

Serves 1

Ingredients:

- 15g parsley
- 15g walnuts
- 15g Parmesan cheese
- 1 tablespoon extra-virgin olive oil
- Juice of ½ lemon
- 50ml water
- 150g skinless chicken breast
- 20g red onions, finely sliced
- 1 teaspoon red wine vinegar
- 35g rocket

- 100g cherry tomatoes, halved
- 1 teaspoon balsamic vinegar

Method:

1. For the pesto, place the parsley, walnuts, Parmesan, olive oil, half the lemon juice and a little water in a blender and whizz to a smooth paste.
2. Marinate the chicken breast in 1 tablespoon of the pesto and the remaining lemon juice in the fridge for 30 minutes.
3. Preheat the oven to 200C.
4. Heat an ovenproof frying pan over medium heat. Fry the chicken for 1 minute on either side, then transfer the pan to the oven and cook for 8 minutes. Spoon another tablespoon of pesto over the chicken. Cover with foil and leave to rest for 5 minutes.
5. Marinate the onions in the red wine vinegar for 5-10 minutes. Drain the liquid.
6. Combine the rocket, tomatoes, and onion and drizzle over the balsamic. Serve with the chicken, spooning over the remaining pesto.

Recipe 12: Blueberry smoothie

Serves 1

Ingredients:

- 1 ripe banana
- 50g blueberries
- 50g blackberries
- 1 tablespoon natural yogurt
- 100ml milk

Method:

1. Blend all the ingredients until smooth.

Recipe 13: Sirtfood Shakshuka

Prep time: 40 minutes

Serves: 1

Ingredients:

- 1 teaspoon extra-virgin olive oil
- 40g red onion, finely chopped
- 1 garlic clove, finely chopped
- 30g celery, finely chopped
- 1 bird's eye chili, finely chopped
- 1 teaspoon ground cumin
- 1 teaspoon ground turmeric
- 1 teaspoon paprika
- 400g tinned chopped tomatoes
- 30g kale, stems removed and roughly chopped

- 1 tablespoon chopped parsley
- 2 medium eggs

Method:

1. Heat a small, deep-sided frying pan over medium-low heat. Add the oil and fry the onion, garlic, celery, chili, and spices for 1–2 minutes.
2. Add the tomatoes, then leave the sauce to simmer gently for 20 minutes, stirring occasionally.
3. Add the kale and cook for a further 5 minutes. If you feel the sauce is getting too thick, simply add a little water. When your sauce has a nice rich consistency, stir in the parsley.
4. Make two little wells in the sauce and crack each egg into them. Reduce the heat to its lowest setting and cover the pan with a lid or foil. Leave the eggs to cook for 10–12 minutes, at which point the whites should be firm while the yolks are still runny. Cook for a further 3–4 minutes if you prefer the yolks to be firm. Serve immediately – ideally straight from the pan.

Recipe 14: Chicken Escalope with sage, caper and parsley and spiced cauliflower 'couscous'

Ingredients:

- 150g cauliflower, roughly chopped

- 1 clove garlic, finely chopped
- 40g red onion, finely chopped
- 1 bird's eye chili, finely chopped
- 1teaspoon fresh ginger, finely chopped
- 2 tablespoon extra-virgin olive oil
- 2 teaspoon ground turmeric
- 30g sun-dried tomatoes, finely chopped
- 10g parsley
- 150g chicken escalope
- 1 teaspoon dried sage
- Juice of ½ lemon
- 1 tablespoon capers

Method:

1. Place the cauliflower in a food processor and pulse in 2-second bursts to finely chop it until it resembles couscous. Set aside.
2. Fry the garlic, red onion, chili and ginger in 1 teaspoon of the oil until soft but not colored.
3. Add the turmeric and cauliflower and cook for 1 minute. Remove from the heat and add the sun-dried tomatoes and half the parsley.
4. Coat the chicken escalope in the remaining oil and sage then fry for 5-6 minutes, turning regularly. When cooked, add the lemon juice, remaining parsley,

capers, and 1 tablespoon water to the pan to make a sauce, then serve.

Recipe 15: Apple Pancakes with Blackcurrant Compote

Prep time 20 minutes

Serves 4

Ingredients:

- 75g porridge oats
- 125g plain flour
- 1 teaspoon baking powder
- 2 tablespoon caster sugar
- Pinch of salt
- 2 apples, peeled, cored and cut into small pieces
- 300ml semi-skimmed milk
- 2 egg whites
- 2 teaspoon light olive oil

For the compote:

- 120g blackcurrants, washed and stalks removed
- 2 tablespoon caster sugar
- 3 tablespoon water

Method:

1. First, make the compote. Place the blackcurrants, sugar, and water in a small pan. Bring up to a simmer and cook for 10-15 minutes.

2. Place the oats, flour, baking powder, caster sugar and salt in a large bowl and mix well. Stir in the apple and then whisk in the milk a little at a time until you have a smooth mixture. Whisk the egg whites to stiff peaks and then fold into the pancake batter. Transfer the batter to a jug.

3. Heat ½ teaspoon oil in a non-stick frying pan on medium-high heat and pour in approximately one-quarter of the batter. Cook on both sides until golden brown. Remove and repeat to make four pancakes.

4. Serve the pancakes with the blackcurrant compote drizzled over.

Recipe 16: Coronation chicken salad

Prep time: 5 minutes

Serves 1

Ingredients:

- 75g natural yogurt
- Juice of ¼ lemon
- 1 teaspoon coriander, chopped
- 1 teaspoon ground turmeric

- ½ teaspoon mild curry powder

- 100g cooked chicken breast, cut into bite-sized pieces

- 6 walnut halves, finely chopped

- 1 medjool date, finely chopped

- 20g red onion, diced

- 1 bird's eye chili

- 40g rocket, to serve

Method:

1. Mix the yogurt, lemon juice, coriander, and spices in a
   bowl. Add all the remaining ingredients and serve on
   a bed of the rocket.

Recipe 17: Prawn Arrabbiata

Prep time 40 minutes

Cook time 30 minutes

Serves 1

Ingredients:

- 125-150g raw or cooked prawns (ideally king prawns)

- 65g buckwheat pasta

- 1 tablespoon extra-virgin olive oil

For Arrabbiata sauce

- 40g red onion, finely chopped
- 1 garlic clove, finely chopped
- 30g celery, finely chopped
- 1 bird's eye chili, finely chopped
- 1 teaspoon dried mixed herbs
- 1 teaspoon extra-virgin olive oil
- 2 tablespoon white wine (optional)
- 400g tinned chopped tomatoes
- 1 tablespoon chopped parsley

Method:

1. Fry the onion, garlic, celery, and chili and dried herbs in the oil over medium-low heat for 1–2 minutes. Turn the heat up to medium, add the wine, and cook for 1 minute. Add the tomatoes and leave the sauce to simmer over medium-low heat for 20–30 minutes, until it has a nice rich consistency. If you feel the sauce is getting too thick simply add a little water.

2. While the sauce is cooking bring a pan of water to the boil and cook the pasta according to the packet instructions. When cooked to your liking, drain, toss with the olive oil and keep in the pan until needed.

3. If you are using raw prawns add them to the sauce and cook for a further 3–4 minutes, until they have turned pink and opaque, add the parsley and serve. If

you are using cooked prawns add them with the parsley, bring the sauce to the boil and serve.

4. Add the cooked pasta to the sauce, mix thoroughly but gently and serve.

Recipe 18: Buckwheat Pasta Salad

Serves 1

Ingredients:

- 50g buckwheat pasta (cooked according to the packet instructions)
- Large handful of rocket
- Small handful of basil leaves
- 8 cherry tomatoes, halved
- ½ avocado, diced
- 10 olives
- 1 tablespoon extra-virgin olive oil
- 20g pine nuts

Method:

1. Gently combine all the ingredients except the pine nuts and arrange on a plate or in a bowl, then scatter the pine nuts over the top.

Recipe 19: Beef Bourguignon stew with mashed potatoes and vegetables

Serves 2

Ingredients:

- 100g streaky bacon diced (or lardons)
- 6 small shallots peeled and chopped in half
- 100g chestnut mushrooms chopped in half (or quarters if really big)
- 400g diced stewing beef
- 1 tablespoon plain flour
- 150ml red wine
- 250ml beef stock from a cube is fine
- 1 bay leaf
- Salt and pepper
- Mashed potatoes and green vegetables to serve or just crusty bread

Method:

1. Preheat the oven to 140C.
2. Put a non-stick frying pan on a medium/high heat and wait a couple of minutes for the pan to heat up. Put the pieces of bacon into the dry pan and fry for 3-4 minutes until really brown and crispy, stirring frequently. Tip the bacon into a large ovenproof dish (it must be one that has a lid).

3. Put the pan back onto the heat and add a drizzle of olive oil and the shallots and mushrooms. Cook for about 3 minutes, stirring frequently until the mushrooms and shallots are a golden brown on both sides. Tip into the ovenproof dish.

4. Put the pan back on the heat and add half the beef. Fry for about 2 minutes on each side until golden brown. Tip into the ovenproof dish and repeat with the other half of the beef.

5. When the second lot of beef is brown, turn down the heat low and sprinkle over the 2 tablespoons of plain flour. Stir to combine, then add the red wine. Bring to the boil, stirring, then tip into the ovenproof dish.

6. Make a quick stock using 2 beef stock cubes and 500ml boiling water. Tip the hot stock into the ovenproof dish and add the bay leaves. Add salt and pepper to taste, then stir the contents of the ovenproof dish so everything is nicely combined. Then put the lid on the dish and put it in the oven for 3 hours.

7. Serve with mashed potatoes and vegetables or crusty bread.

Recipe 20: Kale and Blackcurrant Smoothie

Prep time 3 minutes

Serves 2

Ingredients:

- 2 teaspoon honey
- 1 cup freshly made green tea
- 10 baby kale leaves, stalks removed
- 1 ripe banana
- 40g blackcurrants, washed and stalks removed
- 6 ice cubes

Method:

1. Stir the honey into the warm green tea until dissolved. Blend all the ingredients in a blender until smooth. Serve immediately.

Recipe 21: Waldorf salad

Serves 2

Ingredients:

- 200g celery, roughly chopped
- 100g apple, roughly chopped
- 50g walnuts, roughly chopped
- 1 small red onion, roughly chopped
- 1 head of chicory, chopped
- 10g flat parsley, chopped
- 1 tablespoon capers

- 10g lovage or celery leaves, roughly chopped

For the dressing:

- 1 tablespoon extra-virgin olive oil
- 1 teaspoon balsamic vinegar
- 1 teaspoon Dijon mustard
- Juice of half a lemon

Method:

1. Mix the celery, apple, walnuts, onion, parsley, capers, and lovage/celery in a medium-sized salad bowl and mix.
2. Make the dressing by whisking together the oil, vinegar, mustard, and lemon juice.
3. Drizzle over the salad, mix and serve.

Recipe 22: Chili Con Carne with Buckwheat

Serves 4

Ingredients:

- 1 red onion, finely chopped
- 3 garlic cloves, finely chopped
- 2 bird's eye chilies, finely chopped
- 1 tablespoon extra-virgin olive oil
- 1 tablespoon ground cumin

- 1 tablespoon ground turmeric
- 400g lean minced beef (5 percent fat)
- 150ml red wine
- 1 red pepper, cored, seeds removed and cut into bite-sized pieces
- 2 x 400g tins chopped tomatoes
- 1 tablespoon tomato purée
- 1 tablespoon cocoa powder
- 150g tinned kidney beans
- 300ml beef stock
- 5g coriander, chopped
- 5g parsley, chopped
- 160g buckwheat

Method:

1. In a casserole, fry the onion, garlic, and chili in the oil over medium heat for 2-3 minutes, then add the spices and cook for a minute.
2. Add the minced beef and brown over high heat. Add the red wine and allow it to bubble to reduce it by half.
3. Add the red pepper, tomatoes, tomato purée, cocoa, kidney beans, and stock and leave to simmer for 1 hour.
4. You may have to add a little water to achieve a thick, sticky consistency.
5. Just before serving, stir in the chopped herbs.

6. Meanwhile, cook the buckwheat according to the packet instructions and serve with the chili.

Recipe 23: Blueberry Banana Pancakes with Chunky Apple Compote and Golden Turmeric Latte

Ingredients:

For the Blueberry Banana Pancakes

- 6 bananas
- 6 eggs
- 150g rolled oats
- 2 teaspoon baking powder
- ¼ teaspoon salt
- 25g blueberries

For the Chunky Apple Compote

- 2 apples
- 5 dates (pitted)
- 1 tablespoon lemon juice
- 1/4 teaspoon cinnamon powder
- pinch salt

For the Golden Turmeric Latte

- 3 cups of coconut milk
- 1 teaspoon turmeric powder

- 1 teaspoon cinnamon powder
- 1 teaspoon raw honey
- Pinch of black pepper (increases absorption)
- Tiny piece of fresh, peeled ginger root
- Pinch of cayenne pepper (optional)

Method:

For the blueberry banana pancakes

1. Pop the rolled oats in a high-speed blender and pulse for 1 minute or until an oat flour has formed.
   Tip: make sure your blender is very dry before doing this or else everything will become soggy.
2. Now add the bananas, eggs, baking powder, and salt to the blender and pulse for 2 minutes until a smooth batter forms.
3. Transfer the mixture to a large bowl and fold in the blueberries. Leave to rest for 10 minutes whilst the baking powder activates.
4. To make your pancakes, add a dollop of butter (this helps to make them delicious and crispy!) to your frying pan on medium-high heat. Add a few spoons of the blueberry pancake mix and fry for until nicely golden on the bottom side. Toss the pancake to fry the other side.

For the chunky apple compote

1. Core and rough chop your apples.

2. Pop everything in a food processor, together with 2 tablespoons of water and a pinch of salt. Pulse to form your chunky apple compote.

For the golden turmeric latte

1. Blend all ingredients in a high-speed blender until smooth.

2. Pour into a small pan and heat for 4 minutes over medium heat until hot but not boiling.

3. Enjoy!

Recipe 24: Sirtfood Braised Puy Lentils

Prep time: 50 minutes

Serves: 1

Ingredients:

- 8 cherry tomatoes, halved
- 2 teaspoon extra-virgin olive oil
- 40g red onion, thinly sliced
- 1 garlic clove, finely chopped
- 40g celery, thinly sliced
- 40g carrots, peeled and thinly sliced
- 1 teaspoon paprika
- 1 teaspoon thyme (dry or fresh)

- 75g puy lentils
- 220ml vegetable stock
- 50g kale, roughly chopped
- 1 tablespoon parsley, chopped
- 20g rocket

Method:

1. Heat your oven to 120°C.
2. Put the tomatoes into a small roasting tin and roast in the oven for 35–45 minutes.
3. Heat a saucepan over low–medium heat. Add 1 teaspoon of the olive oil with the red onion, garlic, celery, and carrot and fry for 1–2 minutes, until softened. Stir in the paprika and thyme and cook for a further minute.
4. Rinse the lentils in a fine-meshed sieve and add them to the pan along with the stock. Bring to the boil, then reduce the heat and simmer gently for 20 minutes with a lid on the pan. Stir the pan every 7 minutes or so, adding a little water if the level drops too much.
5. Add the kale and cook for a further 10 minutes. When the lentils are cooked, stir in the parsley and roasted tomatoes. Serve with the rocket drizzled with the remaining teaspoon of olive oil.

Recipe 25: Green Tea Smoothie

Prep time 3 minutes

Serves 2

Ingredients:

- 2 ripe bananas
- 250ml milk
- 2 teaspoon matcha green tea powder
- ½ teaspoon vanilla bean paste (not extract) or a small scrape of the seeds from a vanilla pod
- 6 ice cubes
- 2 teaspoon honey

Method:

1. Simply blend all the ingredients in a blender and serve in two glasses.

Recipe 26: Salmon Sirt Super Salad

Serves 1

Ingredients:

- 50g rocket
- 50g chicory leaves
- 100g smoked salmon slices
- 80g avocado, peeled, stoned and sliced

- 40g celery, sliced

- 20g red onion, sliced

- 15g walnuts, chopped

- 1 tablespoon capers

- 1 large Medjool date, pitted and chopped

- 1 tablespoon extra-virgin olive oil

- Juice of ¼ lemon

- 10g parsley, chopped

- 10g lovage or celery leaves, chopped

Method:

1. Arrange the salad leaves on a large plate. Mix all the remaining ingredients and serve on top of the leaves.

Recipe 27: Chinese-Style Pork with Pak Choi

Serves 4

Ingredients:

- 1 tablespoon extra-virgin olive oil

- 400g firm tofu, cut into large cubes

- 1 tablespoon cornflour

- 1 tablespoon water

- 125ml chicken stock

- 1 tablespoon rice wine

- 1 tablespoon tomato purée

- 1 teaspoon brown sugar
- 1 tablespoon soy sauce
- 1 clove garlic, peeled and crushed
- 1 thumb (5cm) fresh ginger, peeled and grated
- 100g shiitake mushrooms, sliced
- 1 shallot, peeled and sliced
- 200g pak choi or choi sum, cut into thin slices
- 400g pork mince (10% fat)
- 100g beansprouts
- Large handful (20g) parsley, chopped

Method:

1. Lay out the tofu on kitchen paper, cover with more kitchen paper, and set aside.
2. In a small bowl, mix the cornflour and water, removing all lumps. Add the chicken stock, rice wine, tomato purée, brown sugar, and soy sauce. Add the crushed garlic and ginger and stir together.
3. In a wok or large frying pan, heat the oil to a high temperature. Add the shiitake mushrooms and stir-fry for 2–3 minutes until cooked and glossy. Remove the mushrooms from the pan with a slotted spoon and set aside. Add the tofu to the pan and stir-fry until golden on all sides. Remove with a slotted spoon and set aside.

4. Add the shallot and pak choi to the wok, stir-fry for 2 minutes, then add the mince. Cook until the mince is cooked through, then add the sauce, reduce the heat a notch and allow the sauce to bubble round the meat for a minute or two. Add the beansprouts, shiitake mushrooms and tofu to the pan and warm through. Remove from the heat, stir through the parsley and serve immediately.

Recipe 28: Buckwheat Pancakes with Strawberries, Dark Chocolate Sauce and Crushed Walnuts

Makes around 6 to 8 pancakes, depending on the size

Ingredients:

For the pancakes

- 350ml milk
- 150g buckwheat flour
- 1 large egg
- 1 tablespoon extra-virgin olive oil

For the chocolate sauce

- 100g dark chocolate (85% cocoa solids)
- 85ml milk
- 1 tablespoon double cream
- 1 tablespoon extra-virgin olive oil

To serve

- 400g strawberries, hulled and chopped
- 100g walnuts, chopped

Method:

1. To make the pancake batter, place all of the ingredients apart from the olive oil in a blender and blend until you have a smooth batter. It should not be too thick or too runny. (You can store any excess batter in an airtight container for up to 5 days in your fridge. Be sure to mix well before using again.)
2. To make the chocolate sauce, melt the chocolate in a heatproof bowl over a pan of simmering water. Once melted, mix in the milk, whisking thoroughly, and then add the double cream and olive oil. You can keep the sauce warm by leaving the water in the pan simmering on a very low heat until your pancakes are ready.
3. To make the pancakes heat a heavy-bottomed frying pan until it starts to smoke, then add the olive oil.
4. Pour some of the batters into the center of the pan, then tip the excess batter around it until you have covered the whole surface, you may have to add a little more batter to achieve this. You will only need to cook the pancake for 1 minute or so on each side of your pan is hot enough.

5. Once you can see it going brown around the edges
    using a spatula to loosen the pancake around its edge,
    then flip it over. Try to flip in one action to avoid
    breaking it.

6. Cook for a further minute or so on the other side and
    transfer to a plate.

7. Place some strawberries in the center and roll up the
    pancake. Continue until you have made as many
    pancakes as required.

8. Spoon over a generous amount of sauce and sprinkle
    over some chopped walnuts.

9. You may find that your first efforts are too fat or fall
    apart but once you find the consistency of your batter
    that works best for you and you get your technique
    perfected you'll be making them like a professional.
    Practice makes perfect in this case.

Recipe 29: Sesame Chicken Salad

Prep time 12 minutes

Serves 2

Ingredients:

- 1 tablespoon sesame seeds
- 1 cucumber, peeled, halved lengthways, deseeded with
  a teaspoon and sliced

- 100g baby kale, roughly chopped
- 60g pak choi, very finely shredded
- ½ red onion, very finely sliced
- 20g parsley, chopped
- 150g cooked chicken, shredded

For the dressing:

- 1 tablespoon extra-virgin olive oil
- 1 teaspoon sesame oil
- Juice of 1 lime
- 1 teaspoon clear honey
- 2 teaspoon soy sauce

Method:

1. Toast the sesame seeds in a dry frying pan for 2 minutes until lightly browned and fragrant. Transfer to a plate to cool.
2. In a small bowl, mix the olive oil, sesame oil, lime juice, honey, and soy sauce to make the dressing.
3. Place the cucumber, kale, pak choi, red onion, and parsley in a large bowl and gently mix. Pour over the dressing and mix again.
4. Distribute the salad between two plates and top with the shredded chicken. Sprinkle over the sesame seeds just before serving.

Recipe 30: Chickpea, Quinoa and Turmeric Curry

Serves 6

Ingredients:

- 500g new potatoes, halved
- 3 garlic cloves, crushed
- 3 teaspoons ground turmeric
- 1 teaspoon ground coriander
- 1 teaspoon chili flakes or powder
- 1 teaspoon ground ginger
- 400g can of coconut milk
- 1 tablespoon tomato purée
- 400g can of chopped tomatoes
- salt and pepper
- 180g quinoa
- 400g can of chickpeas, drained and rinsed
- 150g spinach

Method:

1. Place the potatoes in a pan of cold water and bring to the boil, then let them cook for about 25 minutes until you can easily stick a knife through them. Drain them well.

2. Place the potatoes in a large pan and add the garlic, turmeric, coriander, chili, ginger, coconut milk, tomato purée, and tomatoes. Bring to the boil, season

with salt and pepper, then add the quinoa with a mug
of just-boiled water (300ml).

3. Reduce the heat to a simmer, place the lid on, and
    allow to cook. Over the next 30 minutes, stirring every
    5 minutes or so to make sure nothing sticks to the
    bottom. Quinoa cooks longer in all these ingredients
    than just in water. Halfway through cooking, add the
    chickpeas. When there are just 5 minutes left, add the
    spinach and stir it in until it wilts. Once the quinoa
    has cooked and is fluffy, not crunchy, it's ready.

BONUS SIRTFOOD DIET RECIPES

BREAKFAST RECIPES

Moroccan Spiced Eggs

Serves 2

Ingredients:

- 1 teaspoon olive oil
- 1 shallot, peeled and finely chopped
- 1 bird's eye chili, deseeded and finely chopped
- 1 garlic clove, peeled and finely chopped
- 1 courgette (zucchini), peeled and finely chopped
- 1 tablespoon tomato puree (paste)
- ½ teaspoon mild chili powder
- ¼ teaspoon ground cinnamon
- ¼ teaspoon ground cumin
- ½ teaspoon salt
- 1 × 400g can chopped tomatoes
- 1 x 400g can chickpeas in water
- Small handful of flat-leaf parsley (10g), chopped
- 4 medium eggs at room temperature

Method:

1. Heat the oil in a saucepan, add the shallot and red (bell) pepper and fry gently for 5 minutes. Then add the garlic and courgette (zucchini) and cook for

another minute or two. Add the tomato puree (paste),
spices, and salt and stir through.

2. Add the chopped tomatoes and chickpeas (soaking
   liquor and all) and increase the heat to medium. With
   the lid off the pan, simmer the sauce for 30 minutes –
   make sure it is gently bubbling throughout and allow
   it to reduce in volume by about one-third.
3. Remove from the heat and stir in the chopped parsley.
4. Preheat the oven to 200C.
5. When you are ready to cook the eggs, bring the
   tomato sauce up to a gentle simmer and transfer it to
   a small oven-proof dish.
6. Crack the eggs on the side of the dish and lower them
   gently into the stew. Cover with foil and bake in the
   oven for 10-15 minutes. Serve the concoction in
   individual bowls with the eggs floating on the top.

Sirtfood Mushroom Scramble Eggs

Ingredients:

- 2 eggs
- 1 teaspoon ground turmeric
- 1 teaspoon mild curry powder
- 20g kale, roughly chopped
- 1 teaspoon extra-virgin olive oil

- ½ bird's eye chili, thinly sliced
- Handful of button mushrooms, thinly sliced
- 5g parsley, finely chopped
- Add a seed mixture as a topper and some Rooster Sauce for flavor (optional)

Method:

1. Mix the turmeric and curry powder and add a little water until you have achieved a light paste.
2. Steam the kale for 2– 3 minutes.
3. Heat the oil in a frying pan over medium heat and fry the chili and mushrooms for 2– 3 minutes until they have started to brown and soften.

Smoked Salmon Omelet

Prep time 10 minutes

Serves 1

Ingredients:

- 2 medium eggs
- 100g smoked salmon, sliced
- ½ teaspoon capers
- 10g rocket, chopped
- 1 teaspoon parsley, chopped
- 1 teaspoon extra-virgin olive oil

Method:

1. Crack the eggs into a bowl and whisk well. Add the salmon, capers, rocket, and parsley.

2. Heat the olive oil in a non-stick frying pan until hot but not smoking. Add the egg mixture and, using a spatula or fish slice, move the mixture around the pan until it is even. Reduce the heat and let the omelet cook through. Slide the spatula around the edges and roll up or fold the omelet in half to serve.

Date and Walnut Porridge

Prep time 10 minutes

Serves 1

Ingredients:

- 200ml milk or dairy-free alternative
- 1 medjool date, chopped
- 35g buckwheat flakes
- 1 teaspoon walnut butter or 4 chopped walnut halves
- 50g strawberries, hulled

Method:

1. Place the milk and date in a pan, heat gently, then add the buckwheat flakes and cook until the porridge is your desired consistency.

2. Stir in the walnut butter or walnuts, top with the strawberries and serve.

Green Omelet

Prep 10 minutes

Serves 1

Ingredients:

- 1 teaspoon olive oil
- 1 shallot, peeled and finely chopped
- 2 large eggs, at room temperature
- 20g rocket leaves
- 10g parsley, finely chopped
- Salt and freshly ground black pepper

Method:

1. In a wide frying pan: heat the oil on medium-low heat and gently fry the shallot for 5 minutes. Turn the heat up a little bit and cook for another 2 minutes.

2. In a bowl or cup, whisk the eggs together well with a fork. Distribute the shallot evenly around the pan before pouring m the eggs. Tip the pan slightly to each

side so that the egg is evenly distributed. Cook for a minute or so before lifting the sides of the omelet and letting any runny egg slip into the base of the pan. Immediately sprinkle over the rocket leaves and parsley and season generously with salt and pepper.

3. When cooked, the top of the omelet will still be soft but not runny and the base will be just starting to brown. Tip onto a plate and enjoy straight away.

Grape and Melon Smoothie

Prep time 2 minutes

Serves 1

Ingredients:

- ½ cucumber, peeled if preferred, halved, seeds removed and roughly chopped
- 30g young spinach leaves, stalks removed
- 100g red seedless grapes
- 100g cantaloupe melon, peeled, deseeded and cut into chunks

Method:

1. Blend in a juicer or blender until smooth.

Chocolate Cupcakes with Matcha Icing

Prep time 35 minutes

Makes 12

Ingredients:

- 150g self-rising flour
- 200g caster sugar
- 60g cocoa
- ½ teaspoon salt
- ½ teaspoon fine espresso coffee, decaf if preferred
- 120ml milk
- ½ teaspoon vanilla extract
- 50ml vegetable oil
- 1 egg
- 120ml boiling water

For the icing:

- 50g butter, at room temperature
- 50g icing sugar
- 1 tablespoon matcha green tea powder
- ½ teaspoon vanilla bean paste
- 50g soft cream cheese

Method:

1. Preheat the oven to 180C.

2. Line a cupcake tin with paper or silicone cake cases.

3. Place the flour, sugar, cocoa, salt, and espresso powder in a large bowl and mix thoroughly.

4. Add the milk, vanilla extract, vegetable oil, and egg to the dry ingredients and use an electric mixer to beat until well combined. Carefully pour in the boiling water slowly and beat on low speed until fully combined. Use high speed to beat for a further minute to add air to the batter. The batter is much more liquid than a normal cake mix. Have faith, it will taste amazing!

5. Spoon the batter evenly between the cake cases. Each cake case should be no more than ¾ full. Bake in the oven for 15-18 minutes, until the mixture bounces back when tapped. Remove from the oven and allow to cool completely before icing.

6. To make the icing, cream the butter and icing sugar together until it's pale and smooth. Add the matcha powder and vanilla and stir again. Finally, add the cream cheese and beat until smooth. Pipe or spread over the cakes.

LUNCH RECIPES

Choc Chip Granola

Prep time 30 minutes

Serves 8

Ingredients:

- 200g jumbo oats
- 50g pecans, roughly chopped
- 3 tablespoon light olive oil
- 20g butter
- 1 tablespoon dark brown sugar
- 2 tablespoon rice malt syrup
- 60g (85%) dark chocolate chips

Method:

1. Preheat the oven to 160°C.
2. Line a large baking tray with a silicone sheet or baking parchment.
3. Mix the oats and pecans in a large bowl. In a small non-stick pan, gently heat the olive oil, butter, brown sugar, and rice malt syrup until the butter has melted and the sugar and syrup have dissolved. Do not allow to boil. Pour the syrup over the oats and stir thoroughly until the oats are fully covered.
4. Distribute the granola over the baking tray, spreading right into the corners. Leave clumps of the mixture with spacing rather than an even spread. Bake in the oven for 20 minutes until just tinged golden brown at

the edges. Remove from the oven and leave to cool on
the tray completely.

5. When cool, break up any bigger lumps on the tray
    with your fingers and then mix in the chocolate chips.
    Scoop or pour the granola into an airtight tub or jar.
    The granola will keep for at least 2 weeks.

Savory Turmeric Pancakes with Lemon Yogurt Sauce

Makes 8 pancakes

Ingredients:

For the yogurt sauce

- 1 cup plain Greek yogurt
- 1 garlic clove, minced
- 1 to 2 tablespoons lemon juice (from 1 lemon), to taste
- ¼ teaspoon ground turmeric
- 10 fresh mint leaves, minced
- 2 teaspoons lemon zest (from 1 lemon)

For the pancakes

- 2 teaspoons ground turmeric
- 1½ teaspoons ground cumin
- 1 teaspoon salt
- 1 teaspoon ground coriander

- ½ teaspoon garlic powder
- ½ teaspoon freshly ground black pepper
- 1 head broccoli, cut into florets
- 3 large eggs, lightly beaten
- 2 tablespoons plain unsweetened almond milk
- 1 cup almond flour
- 4 teaspoons coconut oil

Method:

1. Make the yogurt sauce. Combine the yogurt, garlic, lemon juice, turmeric, mint, and zest in a bowl. Taste and season with more lemon juice, if needed. Set aside or refrigerate until ready to serve.
2. Make the pancakes. In a small bowl, combine the turmeric, cumin, salt, coriander, garlic, and pepper.
3. Place the broccoli in a food processor, and pulse until the florets are broken up into small pieces. Transfer the broccoli to a large bowl and add the eggs, almond milk, and almond flour. Stir in the spice mix and combine well.
4. Heat 1 teaspoon of the coconut oil in a nonstick pan over medium-low heat. Pour ¼ cup batter into the skillet. Cook the pancake until small bubbles begin to appear on the surface and the bottom is golden brown, 2 to 3 minutes. Flip over and cook the pancake for 2 to 3 minutes more. To keep warm, transfer the

cooked pancakes to an oven-safe dish and place it in a 200°F oven.

5. Continue making the remaining 3 pancakes, using the remaining oil and batter.

Buckwheat Noodles with Chicken Kale & Miso Dressing

Prep time 15 minutes

Cook time 15 minutes

Total time 30 minutes

Serves 2

Ingredients:

For the noodles

- 2-3 handfuls of kale leaves (removed from the stem and roughly cut)
- 150g buckwheat noodles (100% buckwheat, no wheat)
- 3-4 shiitake mushrooms, sliced
- 1 teaspoon coconut oil
- 1 red onion, finely diced
- 1 medium free-range chicken breast, sliced or diced
- 1 bird's eye chili, thinly sliced (deseeded if you don't like it hot)

- 2 large garlic cloves, finely diced
- 2-3 tablespoons soy sauce

For the miso dressing

- 1½ tablespoon fresh organic miso
- 1 tablespoon soy sauce
- 1 tablespoon extra-virgin olive oil
- 1 tablespoon lemon or lime juice
- 1 teaspoon sesame oil (optional)

Method:

1. Bring a medium saucepan of water to boil. Add the kale and cook for 1 minute, until slightly wilted. Remove and set aside but reserve the water and bring it back to the boil. Add the buckwheat noodles and cook according to the package instructions (usually about 5 minutes). Rinse under cold water and set aside.

2. In the meantime, pan fry the shiitake mushrooms in a little coconut oil (about a teaspoon) for 2-3 minutes, until lightly browned on each side. Sprinkle with sea salt and set aside.

3. In the same frying pan, heat more coconut oil over medium-high heat. Sauté onion and chili for 2-3 minutes and then add the chicken pieces. Cook 5 minutes over medium heat, stirring a couple of times,

then add the garlic, soy sauce, and a little splash of water. Cook for a further 2-3 minutes, stirring frequently until chicken is cooked through.

4. Finally, add the kale and buckwheat noodles and toss through the chicken to warm up.

5. Mix the miso dressing and drizzle over the noodles right at the end of cooking, this way you will keep all those beneficial probiotics in the miso alive and active.

Baked Salmon Salad with Creamy Mint Dressing

Prep time 20 minutes

Serves 1

Ingredients:

- 1 salmon fillet (130g)
- 40g mixed salad leaves
- 40g young spinach leaves
- 2 radishes, trimmed and thinly sliced
- 5cm piece (50g) cucumber, cut into chunks
- 2 spring onions, trimmed and sliced
- 1 small handful (10g) parsley, roughly chopped

For the dressing:

- 1 teaspoon low-fat mayonnaise

- 1 tablespoon natural yogurt
- 1 tablespoon rice vinegar
- 2 leaves mint, finely chopped
- Salt and freshly ground black pepper

Method:

1. Preheat the oven to 200°C.
2. Place the salmon fillet on a baking tray and bake for 16–18 minutes until just cooked through. Remove from the oven and set aside. The salmon is equally nice hot or cold in the salad. If your salmon has skin, simply cook skin side down and remove the salmon from the skin using a fish slice after cooking. It should slide off easily when cooked.
3. In a small bowl, mix the mayonnaise, yogurt, rice wine vinegar, mint leaves, and salt and pepper and leave to stand for at least 5 minutes to allow the flavors to develop.
4. Arrange the salad leaves and spinach on a serving plate and top with the radishes, cucumber, spring onions, and parsley. Flake the cooked salmon onto the salad and drizzle the dressing over.

Fragrant Asian Hotpot

Prep time 15 minutes

Serves 2

Ingredients:

- 1 teaspoon tomato purée
- 1 star anise, crushed (or ¼ teaspoon ground anise)
- Small handful (10g) parsley, stalks finely chopped
- Small handful (10g) coriander, stalks finely chopped
- Juice of ½ lime
- 500ml chicken stock, fresh or made with 1 cube
- ½ carrot, peeled and cut into matchsticks
- 50g broccoli, cut into small florets
- 50g beansprouts
- 100g raw tiger prawns
- 100g firm tofu, chopped
- 50g rice noodles, cooked according to packet instructions
- 50g cooked water chestnuts, drained
- 20g sushi ginger, chopped
- 1 tablespoon good-quality miso paste

Method:

1. Place the tomato purée, star anise, parsley stalks, coriander stalks, lime juice, and chicken stock in a large pan and bring to a simmer for 10 minutes.
2. Add the carrot, broccoli, prawns, tofu, noodles, and water chestnuts and simmer gently until the prawns

are cooked through. Remove from the heat and stir in the sushi ginger and miso paste.

3. Serve sprinkled with the parsley and coriander leaves.

Lamb, Butternut Squash and Date Tagine

Prep time 15 minutes

Cook time 1 hour 15 minutes

Total time 1 hour 30 minutes

Serves 4

Ingredients:

- 2 tablespoons olive oil
- 1 red onion, sliced
- 2cm ginger, grated
- 3 garlic cloves, grated or crushed
- 1 teaspoon chili flakes (or to taste)
- 2 teaspoons cumin seeds
- 1 cinnamon stick
- 2 teaspoons ground turmeric
- 800g lamb neck fillet, cut into 2cm chunks
- ½ teaspoon salt
- 100g medjool dates, pitted and chopped
- 400g tin chopped tomatoes, plus half a can of water

- 500g butternut squash, chopped into 1cm cubes
- 400g tin chickpeas, drained
- 2 tablespoons fresh coriander (plus extra for garnish)
- 300g buckwheat

Method:

1. Preheat the oven to 140C.
2. Drizzle about 2 tablespoons of olive oil into a large ovenproof saucepan or cast iron casserole dish. Add the sliced onion and cook on a gentle heat, with the lid on, for about 5 minutes, until the onions are softened but not brown.
3. Add the grated garlic and ginger, chili, cumin, cinnamon, and turmeric. Stir well and cook for 1 more minute with the lid off. Add a splash of water if it gets too dry.
4. Add in the lamb chunks. Stir well to coat the meat in the onions and spices and then add the salt, chopped dates, and tomatoes, plus about half a can of water (100-200ml).
5. Bring the tagine to the boil and then put the lid on and put in the preheated oven for 1 hour and 15 minutes.
6. 30 minutes before the end of the cooking time, add in the chopped butternut squash and drained chickpeas. Stir everything together, put the lid back on and return to the oven for the final 30 minutes of cooking.

7. When the tagine is ready, remove from the oven and stir through the chopped coriander. Serve with buckwheat already cooked according to the packet instruction.

Note:

If you don't own an ovenproof saucepan or cast iron casserole dish, simply cook the tagine in a regular saucepan up until it has to go in the oven and then transfer the tagine into a regular lidded casserole dish before placing in the oven. Add on an extra 5 minutes of cooking time to allow for the fact that the casserole dish will need extra time to heat up.

Turmeric Baked Salmon

Prep time 15 minutes

Cook time 10 minutes

Serves 1

Ingredients:

- 150g skinned salmon
- 1 teaspoon extra-virgin olive oil
- 1 teaspoon ground turmeric
- Juice of ¼ lemon

For the spicy celery:

- 1 teaspoon extra-virgin olive oil
- 40g red onion, finely chopped
- 60g tinned green lentils
- 1 garlic clove, finely chopped
- 1 cm fresh ginger, finely chopped
- 1 Bird's eye chili, finely chopped
- 150g celery, cut into 2cm lengths
- 1 teaspoon mild curry powder
- 130g tomato, cut into 8 wedges
- 100ml chicken or vegetable stock
- 1 tablespoon chopped parsley

Method:

1. Heat the oven to 200C.
2. Start with the spicy celery. Heat a frying pan over medium-low heat, add the olive oil, then the onion, garlic, ginger, chili, and celery. Fry gently for 2–3 minutes or until softened but not colored, then add the curry powder and cook for a further minute.
3. Add the tomatoes then the stock and lentils and simmer gently for 10 minutes. You may want to increase or decrease the cooking time depending on how crunchy you like your celery.

4. Meanwhile, mix the turmeric, oil, and lemon juice and rub over the salmon.

5. Place on a baking tray and cook for 8–10 minutes.

6. To finish, stir the parsley through the celery and serve with the salmon.

Greek Salad Skewers

Prep time 10 minutes

Serves 2

Ingredients:

- 2 wooden skewers, soaked in water for 30 minutes before use
- 8 large black olives
- 8 cherry tomatoes
- 1 yellow pepper, cut into 8 squares
- ½ red onion, cut in half and separated into 8 pieces
- 100g (about 10cm) cucumber, cut into 4 slices and halved
- 100g feta, cut into 8 cubes

For the dressing:

- 1 tablespoon extra-virgin olive oil
- Juice of ½ lemon
- 1 teaspoon balsamic vinegar

- ½ clove garlic, peeled and crushed
- Few leaves basil, finely chopped (or ½ teaspoon dried mixed herbs to replace basil and oregano)
- Few leaves oregano, finely chopped
- Generous seasoning of salt and freshly ground black pepper

Method:

1. Thread each skewer with the salad ingredients in the order: olive, tomato, yellow pepper, red onion, cucumber, feta, tomato, olive, yellow pepper, red onion, cucumber, feta.
2. Place all the dressing ingredients in a small bowl and mix thoroughly. Pour over the skewers.

DINNER RECIPES

Kale, Edamame and Tofu Curry

Prep time 45 minutes

Serves 4

Ingredients:

- 1 tablespoon extra-virgin olive oil
- 1 large red onion, chopped
- 4 cloves garlic, peeled and grated

- 1 large thumb (7cm) fresh ginger, peeled and grated
- 1 bird's eye chili, deseeded and thinly sliced
- ½ teaspoon ground turmeric
- ¼ teaspoon cayenne pepper
- 1 teaspoon paprika
- ½ teaspoon ground cumin
- 1 teaspoon salt
- 250g dried red lentils
- 1 liter boiling water
- 50g frozen soya edamame beans
- 200g firm tofu, chopped into cubes
- 2 tomatoes, roughly chopped
- Juice of 1 lime
- 200g kale leaves, stalks removed and torn

Method:

1. Put the oil in a heavy-bottomed pan over low-medium heat. Add the onion and cook for 5 minutes before adding the garlic, ginger, and chili and cooking for a further 2 minutes. Add the turmeric, cayenne, paprika, cumin, and salt. Stir through before adding the red lentils and stirring again.

2. Pour in the boiling water and bring to a hearty simmer for 10 minutes, then reduce the heat and cook

for a further 20-30 minutes until the curry has a thick 'porridge' consistency.

3. Add the soya beans, tofu, and tomatoes and cook for a further 5 minutes. Add the lime juice and kale leaves and cook until the kale is just tender.

Baked Potatoes with Spicy Chickpea Stew

Prep time 10 minutes

Cook time 1 hour

Serves 4-6

Ingredients:

- 4-6 baking potatoes, pricked all over
- 2 tablespoons extra-virgin olive oil
- 2 red onions, finely chopped
- 4 cloves garlic, grated or crushed
- 2cm ginger, grated
- ½ -2 teaspoons chili flakes (depending on how hot you like things)
- 2 tablespoons cumin seeds
- 2 tablespoons turmeric
- Splash of water
- 2 x 400g tins chopped tomatoes
- 2 tablespoons unsweetened cocoa powder (or cacao)

- 2 x 400g tins chickpeas (or kidney beans if you prefer) including the chickpea water DON'T DRAIN!!
- 2 yellow peppers (or whatever color you prefer!), chopped into bite-size pieces
- 2 tablespoons parsley plus extra for garnish
- Salt and pepper to taste (optional)
- Side salad (optional)

Method:

1. Preheat the oven to 200C.
2. When the oven is hot enough put the baking potatoes in the oven and cook for 1 hour or until they are done how you like them.
3. Once the potatoes are in the oven, place the olive oil and chopped red onion in a large wide saucepan and cook gently, with the lid on for 5 minutes, until the onions are soft but not brown.
4. Remove the lid and add the garlic, ginger, cumin, and chili. Cook for a further minute on low heat, then add the turmeric and a very small splash of water and cook for another minute, taking care not to let the pan get too dry.
5. Add in the tomatoes, cocoa powder (or cacao), chickpeas (including the chickpea water), and yellow pepper. Bring to the boil, then simmer on a low heat for 45 minutes until the sauce is thick and unctuous

(but don't let it burn!). The stew should be done at roughly the same time as the potatoes.

6. Finally stir in the 2 tablespoons of parsley, and some salt and pepper if you wish, and serve the stew on top of the baked potatoes, perhaps with a simple side salad.

Chicken Korma

Ingredients:

- 2 tablespoons extra-virgin olive oil
- 1 red onion, sliced
- 750g skinless chicken breast or thigh chopped into 2cm chunks
- 2 cm piece of ginger, grated
- 2 garlic cloves, grated or crushed
- 1 teaspoon turmeric
- 2 teaspoons garam masala
- 400ml tin coconut milk
- 3 tablespoons ground almonds
- 1 tablespoon coriander chopped (plus extra for garnish)

Method:

1. Put the olive oil in a wide, deep saucepan and add the sliced onions. Cook on low heat, covered with a lid, for 5 minutes until the onions are soft but not brown.

2. Take the lid off and add the chunks of chicken. Turn the heat up to medium-high and cook for 5 minutes until golden brown, stirring occasionally.

3. Turn the heat down and add the grated ginger and garlic together with the turmeric and garam masala. Cook for 2 minutes, stirring occasionally.

4. Add about ¾ of the coconut milk, bring to the boil and then turn down and gently simmer for 10 minutes. If you find the curry becomes too dry you can add the rest of the coconut milk.

5. After 10 minutes, add the ground almonds and chopped coriander and cook for 1 more minute, then serve with rice and garnish with a little more chopped coriander.

Easy Peasy Coq au Vin

Prep time 5 minutes

Cook time 40 minutes

Total time 45 minutes

Serves 4

Ingredients:

- 1 tablespoon extra-virgin olive oil
- 1 red onion, chopped
- 600g boneless, skinless chicken thighs
- 200ml French red wine (such as Cotes du Rhone)
- 200ml chicken stock
- 2 bay leaves
- 2 sprigs thyme
- Salt and pepper
- 90g lardons (or chopped up smoked bacon)
- 100g chestnut mushrooms roughly chopped
- 400g new potatoes to serve
- Green vegetables to serve

Method:

1. Place the oil and onions in a large saucepan or flameproof casserole dish and cook gently over a medium/low heat for 3 minutes until softened.
2. Turn up the heat and add the chicken thigh fillets. Cook for 3 minutes, stirring occasionally until the thigh fillets are slightly browned.
3. Add the wine and stock, plus the bay leaves and thyme, and bring to the boil. Turn down and put the lid on.

4. Next, put a non-stick frying pan on a high heat and wait for 1 minute. Then tip in the lardons and cook, stirring frequently for 1 minute, before adding in the mushrooms and cooking for a further 2 minutes. The lardons should be golden and the mushrooms nicely browned. Tip the lardons and mushrooms into the chicken stew and stir everything. Replace the lid and continue cooking the stew for 15 minutes.

5. After 15 minutes, remove the lid. Stir the casserole and then leave the lid off to allow the sauce to thicken slightly (see note 1). Continue cooking for a further 15 minutes or until your potatoes and green veggies are cooked.

6. While your stew is cooking boil or steam your new potatoes for 15 minutes and steam your green veg for 5 minutes (or longer if you prefer them softer).

7. Serve the Coq au Vin with the new potatoes, green veg and a glass of the same wine you used in the stew.

Note:

This stew produces a thin French style 'jus' rather than a thick English gravy. If you'd prefer a thicker gravy, mix 1 teaspoon flour or cornflour with a very small amount of water and then add this mixture to the stew when you add the lardons and mushrooms.

Quick Beany Chili

Prep time 5 minutes

Cook time 20 minutes

Total time 25 minutes

Serves 4

Ingredients:

- 200g brown rice
- 1 red onion, sliced thinly
- 1 tablespoon extra-virgin olive oil
- 3 garlic cloves, crushed or finely chopped
- ½ teaspoon chili or more if you like it hot!
- 1 teaspoon cumin seeds, ground
- 1 teaspoon paprika
- 2 x 400g tins chopped tomatoes
- Salt and pepper
- 1 x 400g tin kidney beans drained
- 1 x 400g tin pinto beans drained
- 2 limes
- 1 tablespoon coriander leaves chopped (plus extra for garnish)
- 1 quantity Easy Peasy Guacamole or 1 pot shop-bought guacamole

Method:

1. Put the 200g brown rice in a saucepan together with 3 times as much boiling water (the easiest way to do this is to find a mug that roughly holds 200g rice and then refill it 3 times for the water) and a pinch of salt.

2. Put a lid on the rice and bring it to the boil, then turn down and simmer for 20 minutes. After 20 minutes, turn the rice off and leave covered for 5 minutes before serving. The rice should have absorbed all the water, but if there is any left, drain it in a sieve.

3. While the rice is cooking put the sliced red onion in a large, wide saucepan and add the extra-virgin olive oil. Put a lid on and gently cook for 5 minutes on low heat, stirring occasionally, until the onions have softened.

4. Add the garlic, chili, cumin, and paprika and cook for one more minute without a lid.

5. Add the tins of tomatoes plus some salt and pepper and bring to the boil, then turn down the heat and simmer uncovered for 10 minutes.

6. After 10 minutes add the 2 tins of drained beans and cook for 5 more minutes. Turn off the heat and then add the juice of one of the limes and 1 tablespoonful of chopped coriander and stir. Cut the other lime into 4 wedges.

7. Scatter the chili with more coriander and serve with the brown rice, lime wedges, and guacamole.

Chicken Fajitas

Prep time 5 minutes

Cook time 10 minutes

Total time 15 minutes

Serves 4

Ingredients:

- 12 flour tortilla wraps
- 2 teaspoons cumin
- 1 teaspoon cayenne pepper (add more if you like things hot)
- 2 teaspoons dried oregano
- Juice of 1 lime
- 2 cloves garlic, grated or crushed
- 2 large chicken breasts, sliced into thin strips
- 2 large red onions, thinly sliced
- 3 bell peppers, sliced into strips (preferably use green, red and yellow)
- 3 tablespoon extra-virgin olive oil
- 2 tablespoons fresh coriander chopped finely

- Your choice of guacamole/sour cream/salsa/grated cheese/extra limes & coriander/tortilla chips to serve - any or all of them!

Method:

1. If you are making your guacamole or salsa, make these first and refrigerate until needed – or ask someone else to make these for you while you get on with the fajitas.
2. Preheat the oven to 200C.
3. Remove the tortilla wraps from the packet and wrap it in foil.
4. Mix the cumin, cayenne pepper, oregano, lime juice, and crushed garlic in a large bowl.
5. Slice the chicken into thin strips and place in the marinade. Toss the chicken to thoroughly coat in the marinade and set aside for 5 minutes (or put in the fridge and marinate for longer if you prefer).
6. Use the time while the chicken is marinating to slice the onions and peppers.
7. When the oven has heated up, put the tortilla wraps in the oven for 8 minutes until warmed through. After 8 minutes remove from the oven but keep wrapped in foil until needed.
8. Stir fry the onions and peppers in a little olive oil on a low heat for 5 minutes until softened but not brown.

Turn up the heat and add the chicken and marinade and fry for about 5 minutes until the chicken is cooked through and browned and the veg is slightly charred.

9. To check if the chicken is cooked all the way through, choose the thickest piece of chicken and cut it in half – if it is completely white with no pink, it is cooked. And if the thickest piece is cooked, so should all the thinners ones!

10. Sprinkle the chicken with the chopped coriander and serve in the pan on the table, together with the warm tortilla wraps and whatever extras you have chosen for people to make up their fajitas. Enjoy!

Soy, Chili and Ginger Salmon

Prep time 5 minutes

Cook time 10 minutes

Total time 15 minutes

Serves 4

Ingredients:

- 6 tablespoons soy sauce
- Juice of 1 lime
- 2 tablespoons sesame oil

- 1 red chili, sliced and seeds removed (plus extra for garnish)
- 2cm ginger, chopped in thin slices (plus extra for garnish)
- 4 salmon fillets
- 200g rice
- 400ml boiling water
- Salt
- Tender stem broccoli
- Pack choi, cut into quarters lengthways
- Vegetable sunflower or wok oil
- Sesame seeds for garnish optional

Method:

1. Mix the soy sauce, lime juice, sesame oil, sliced chili, and ginger in a bowl to make a simple marinade.
2. Cut each salmon fillet into 4 equal chunks and put it into the marinade. Turn the salmon pieces over a few times to coat them in the marinade and set aside.
3. Next put the rice at the bottom of a steamer and add the water and salt. Put the prepared vegetables in the top of the steamer and place over the rice. Bring the rice to the boil and turn down very low. Cook for 8 minutes, by which time the rice should be just cooked and should have absorbed all the water and the vegetables should be just done.

4. While the rice and the vegetables are cooking, drizzle a little oil into a frying pan and heat over medium heat for 1 minute. Add the salmon, reserving the marinade for later. Cook the salmon for about 3 minutes on each side (top and bottom sides, not all the sides!) and then turn the heat down and tip in the marinade. Cook for a further 2 minutes.

5. Sprinkle the salmon with a few sesame seeds and some extra chili and ginger and serve with the rice and green vegetables. I like to put the soy sauce and a few limes on the table for everyone to help themselves to extra.

Buckwheat Bean and Tomato Risotto

Serves 4

Ingredients:

- 2 tablespoon extra-virgin olive oil
- 2 cloves of garlic, chopped
- 225g buckwheat
- 400ml of hot water or vegetable stock
- 225g frozen broad beans
- ½ cup of sun-dried tomatoes in oil
- Juice of ½ lemon
- 2 tablespoon coriander, chopped

- 50g almonds, toasted
- Salt and pepper

Method:

1. Heat the olive oil in a frying pan. Add the garlic and cook for a minute.
2. Add the buckwheat to the pan and stir it well to coat it in the oil.
3. Add the hot water or stock. Cover and simmer for 10 minutes.
4. Stir in the broad beans. Cook for a few minutes until the beans are just tender.
5. Add the sun-dried tomatoes, lemon juice, fresh herbs and almonds and season with salt and pepper.